Victor Manuel Sanchez Castillo

Liposuction

AF301905

Victor Manuel Sanchez Castillo

Liposuction

Complications and prevention

ScienciaScripts

Imprint
Any brand names and product names mentioned in this book are subject to trademark, brand or patent protection and are trademarks or registered trademarks of their respective holders. The use of brand names, product names, common names, trade names, product descriptions etc. even without a particular marking in this work is in no way to be construed to mean that such names may be regarded as unrestricted in respect of trademark and brand protection legislation and could thus be used by anyone.

Cover image: www.ingimage.com

This book is a translation from the original published under ISBN 978-613-9-68150-1.

Publisher:
Sciencia Scripts
is a trademark of
Dodo Books Indian Ocean Ltd. and OmniScriptum S.R.L publishing group

120 High Road, East Finchley, London, N2 9ED, United Kingdom
Str. Armeneasca 28/1, office 1, Chisinau MD-2012, Republic of Moldova, Europe
Printed at: see last page
ISBN: 978-620-8-19436-9

Copyright © Victor Manuel Sanchez Castillo
Copyright © 2024 Dodo Books Indian Ocean Ltd. and OmniScriptum S.R.L publishing group

Summary:

Thank you: 2
Summary: 3
Introduction: 4
METHOD 9
Results and discussion: 10
Conclusion: 37
ANNEXES 38
Bibliographical references: 45

<u>**Thanks:**</u>

To my family: my wife Cary and daughters Roxanna and Rosangela, for their patience and understanding so that I could complete my postgraduate course, for the time I didn't dedicate, for the days I was away from you: thank you.

To the Coordinator Prof. Dr. Eduardo Teixeira and the teachers of the Aesthetic Plastic Surgery Postgraduate Course, for the knowledge acquired and the professionalism demonstrated, for the ethics and good treatment, to all: thank you.

<u>Summary:</u>

Liposuction, like any surgical procedure, has inherent risks. The plastic surgeon must have a thorough understanding of its problems, prevention and management. Proper patient selection, careful medical records, imaging, consent, information, anesthesiologist, pre-operative evaluation and standardized surgical technique, strict evaluation, replacement fluid, also including lidocaine, infiltration, trans. and post-operative control factors, are helping to reduce complications related to liposuction.

Liposuction performed for aesthetic procedures aims to remove fat in healthy patients and reduce the accumulation of localized fat, known as lipodystrophy, leading to an improvement in body contour. Over the last three decades, liposuction has been perfected; however, like any other surgical procedure, it is not without its complications. The aim of this study is to review the bibliography using Pubmed, identifying complications after liposuction and their prevention.

Key words: Liposuction. Post-operative complications. Embolism. Prevention.

Introduction:

Liposuction went from being a novelty in the late 1970s to becoming the most common procedure performed by plastic surgeons in the last decade. Dujarrier in 1921 was the first to use a cannula to remove adipose tissue for aesthetic reasons, with a disastrous result. Interest in fat removal using small cannulas resurfaced in the 1960s when Schrudde used sharp curettes with negative pressure for fat removal. In the 1980s, blunt cannulas were introduced and at the end of this decade Klein presented the tumescent technique which minimizes fluid loss. In 1992, Zocchi revolutionized the technique with the help of ultrasound (1,2).

Liposuction was described by Gerard Illouz in 1977 with the aim of treating lipodystrophy (1, 2). Liposuction has been integrated into the plastic surgeon's therapeutic arsenal through studies and surgical practice. Scientific studies have certified the indications, limitations and complications of this technique, making it safe to use (2, 3).

However, the breadth of the areas to be treated often makes it difficult to analyze perioperative results (3). Turning this assessment into numbers doesn't put an end to personal interpretations by surgeons and patients, but it does allow for a less subjective demonstration.

Liposuction, performed as an aesthetic procedure to remove fat in healthy patients, aims to reduce the accumulation of localized fat, known as lipodystrophy, leading to an improvement in body contour. Over the last three decades, liposuction has been improved, reducing the invasiveness of the surgery and preserving local circulation (1,2). According to statistics from the American Society of Plastic Surgeons (ASPS), around 198,000 individuals underwent liposuction in 2009 in the United States(3), placing it fourth among the five most common aesthetic procedures. The Brazilian Society of Plastic Surgery (SBCP)(3), which is among the largest plastic surgery organizations in the world, reports, in conjunction with a survey by the Datafolha Institute, that 629,000 plastic surgeries are performed every year in Brazil, 73% of which are cosmetic and 27% restorative. Among these aesthetic surgical procedures, 20% are represented by liposuction, second only to breast augmentation, meaning that more than 90,000 liposuction surgeries are performed in the country every year (4). However, like any other surgical procedure, liposuction is not without its local or systemic complications. Among the many local complications are skin irregularities (visible and palpable), prolonged edema, bruising, hyperpigmentation, changes in skin sensitivity, seromas, hematomas, insufficient correction of lipodystrophy, skin ulcers and necrosis, local infections, contact dermatitis, unsightly scars and persistent edema. Among the systemic complications of classic liposuction are visceral perforations, allergic reactions to medications during and after surgery, febrile reactions, systemic infections, cardiac arrhythmias, tachycardia, anemia, hypovolemic shock, pulmonary thromboembolism and deep vein thrombosis, fat embolism, fat embolism syndrome, sepsis and even death (4-5). Invariably, the media and the public in general massively publicize cases of complications, especially those of greater severity.

The aim of this study was to review the literature using PubMed, identifying complications following classic liposuction, including only those performed for aesthetic purposes.

To better understand the liposuction process, we have included a brief review of the histology of the hypodermis, also called subcutaneous tissue, or superficial fascia, which is the lowest layer of the integumentary system in vertebrates. The types of cells found in the hypodermis are fibroblasts, fat cells and macrophages. It derives from the mesoderm but, unlike the dermis, does not result from the dermatome region of the mesoderm. The hypodermis is mainly used to store fat (6).

Composition:

Its collagen and elastic fibers connect directly with those of the dermis and run in all directions, although mainly parallel to the surface of the skin. Where the skin is very flexible, the fibers are scarce; instead, where it adheres to the underlying parts (palmar and plantar regions), they are thick and numerous.

Depending on the regions of the body and the body's nutrition, a varying number of fat cells develop in the subcutaneous layer. These cells can reach a thickness in the abdomen of 3 cm or more, but in other areas such as the penis and eyelids, the subcutaneous layer contains no fat cells.

The subcutaneous layer is crossed by numerous blood vessels and nerve trunks; they contain many nerve endings.

The subcutaneous tissue is divided into the superficial areolar layer and the deep lamellar or reticular layer. The lamellar layer is more susceptible to an increase in thickness in cases of fat accumulation. The number of fat cells present in the lamellar layer is the main cause of hypertrophy and an increase in the thickness of the panniculus adiposus, with one fat cell being able to grow up to a hundred times its original volume. Subcutaneous cellular tissue behaves differently in certain areas of the body. Body regions where the skin is thicker and firmer, such as the chest, show greater development of the areolar layer to the detriment of the lamellar layer (7,8).

Layers:

Areolar

It is the outermost layer and is in contact with the dermis, formed by adipocytes.

Lamellar

This is the deepest layer, the cells are spindle-shaped, small and horizontally distributed; this layer increases when people gain weight, due to the increase in the volume of adipocytes capable of invading the most superficial layer of the skin.

Functions of the hypodermic (7):

It helps maintain the body's temperature, gives shape to the body's contour and provides mobility to the skin as a whole. Its thickness can change depending on the parts of the body and can differ from person to person.

The lymphatic system plays an important role in the self-cleansing of the skin. The articulated vessels run parallel to the blood lymph circulating between the skin and muscles.

Adipose cells or adipocytes are cells that store fat and regulate body temperature.

Adipocytes are cells that form part of adipose tissue and are responsible for storing fat in the human body. Each fat cell stores a certain amount of fat. They are capable of storing fat up to ten times their size. When the storage limit of a fat cell is exceeded, a new cell is created in the adipose tissue. Adipose tissue accompanies human development throughout life. (1)

First of all, we should know that fat storage cells are called adipocytes and from a weight loss point of view, the important thing is to understand how the fat is removed from the adipocyte and used by the muscles involved in the exercise (7,8). The idea that I'm going to do 500 sit-ups to lose belly fat doesn't exist, because the fat isn't burned where the exercise is taking place. The fat stored in the adipocyte is in the form of triglycerides (three fatty acids linked to a glycerol molecule). While exercising, various hormones such as catecholamines, glucagon, growth hormone, corticosteroids, among others, are released into the bloodstream, and when they reach the adipocytes, they cause lipolysis (breakdown of triglycerides) increasing blood concentrations of free fatty acids (FFA). These FFA are taken to the skeletal muscles which use them to synthesize ATP. The fatty acid, now inside the muscle cell, needs to be activated (incorporation of Acyl-CoA) and transported into the mitochondrial matrix, where it will be broken down into two-carbon molecules (Acetyl-CoA) to be oxidized (Beta-oxidation). Inside the mitochondria, the Acetyl-CoA molecules are processed in the citric acid cycle (Krebs Cycle) and produce NADH and FADH2. The latter are transferred to the electron transport chain where ATP is finally generated. FADH2 gives rise to 2 ATP, while NADH gives rise to 3 ATP. From the point of view of energy generation, glucose and fatty acids are the most important substrates. The complete oxidation of 1g of glucose generates approximately 4 Kcal, while the same amount of fatty acids (fat) generates around 9 Kcal.(1)

Adipocytes are highly specialized cells whose function is to balance the body's energy flow by storing energy in the form of fat (lipids) when calorie intake is higher than consumption and releasing energy (in the form of fatty acids) during periods of low calorie intake.

The fat reservoir occupies almost the entire cytoplasm of the adipocyte. A mature adipocyte has around 80-95% fat in its volume, which can correspond to 0.5-1µg of fat per cell. In order to store this amount of lipids, adipocytes can increase their diameter by around 20 times and vary their volume by hundreds of times. It is estimated that an adult individual stores between 10 and 20 kg of body fat in their adipocytes, which corresponds to 90,000 - 180,000 kcal, enough to live on fasted food for around 45-90 days.

Most adipose tissue develops during the period close to birth, but the number of adipocytes can increase according to diet and calorie intake during life.

There are two types of mature adipocytes with different morphology, distribution and physiology: unilocular and multilocular adipocytes (7).

Unilocular adipocytes have only a single large inclusion of lipid in their cytoplasm and their main function is to store energy when there is an increase in calorie intake and to provide energy during periods of fasting or a shortage of calories. In humans, this cell type is distributed throughout the subcutaneous surface of the body and in the abdominal region. Unilocular adipocytes are originally spherical, but can be polygonal in shape due to the mutual deformation caused by their increased volume and subsequent pressure. The size of a unilocular adipocyte varies between 20-200nm in diameter and the amount of lipids stored inside can vary between 60 and 85% of its total weight. Due to the large inclusion of lipid in its cytoplasm, the nucleus and all the other organelles are displaced to the cell periphery.

Multilocular adipocytes get their name from having several lipid inclusions in their cytoplasm and their main function is to supply energy in the form of heat. Their location is limited to specific regions. In newborns, multilocular adipocyte deposits are found in the cervical, axillary, supra-iliac and perirenal regions. They vary in shape and can be found in spherical, fusiform or polygonal form. Their cytoplasm contains numerous lipid inclusions and their nucleus is, as in unilocular adipocytes, displaced towards the cytoplasmic periphery.

The key to successful liposuction begins with proper patient selection, a thorough medical history that assesses history and risk factors, and open communication about the procedure, including its risks, complications and limitations.

Although liposuction is considered a safe procedure, it does have some inherent risks, which in most cases can be avoided with meticulous surgical technique and careful pre-operative analysis.

Liposuction is undoubtedly one of the most widely performed surgical procedures in the world, either on its own, in association with other surgeries or as a complement to other treatments. However, its apparent simplicity has led many surgeons to make serious mistakes, either because they underestimate the risks or because they are unfamiliar with the technique in all its aspects and details.

As a complicating factor, it is often presented in an absurdly unethical way in the media. It is often presented as a magic solution for weight loss, as a surgery free of complications, as a procedure so simple that it can be carried out with impunity in offices or environments totally devoid of the minimum safety resources. All this means that bad results multiply and complications become more and more serious. Many doctors from other specialties view liposuction with suspicion and even contempt, formally refusing to recommend it. Many potential patients refuse to undergo liposuction because they see it as "too dangerous".

The articles reviewed describe tactics aimed at greater perioperative control of liposuction, associated with a reduction in complaints and postoperative complications related to possible asymmetries and hypocorrections in the treated areas.

With the review of the literature we investigated the different factors that influence post-operative evolution, risk factors, the pathophysiological elements that interact, the characteristics of the different procedures, and the preventive and therapeutic schedule of different authors, specifically related to complications and how to obtain an aesthetic and functional result with prompt recovery of the patient.

METHOD

A search was carried out on the MEDLINE/PubMed database, evaluating all published articles that referred to complications in liposuction for aesthetic purposes, whether or not associated with other surgical procedures. The expressions used in this *online* search were: *"complication after liposuction" "complication in liposuction" "fat embolism after liposuction" "fat embolism following liposuction"* and *"deaths related to liposuction"*.After this survey, the articles were divided, according to the characteristics of the publication, into: case reports, experimental studies, and complications in liposuction isolated or associated with other procedures. Fifty-four articles of interest were found, and all repeated, irrelevant or out of line with the research proposal were excluded.

We found 84 articles using the expression *"complication in liposuction",* 56 articles with *"complication after liposuction",* 27 articles with *"fat embolism after liposuction"*, 7 articles with *"fat embolism following liposuction"* and 16 articles with *"deaths related to liposuction"*. Of these articles, only 84 were considered related to the subject, with cases of fat embolism after liposuction, visceral perforation, vascular injury, blindness and herpes zoster infection being found, among other reports. Based on the articles analyzed, it was possible to conclude that liposuction is a highly effective procedure when well indicated and well performed, but there are risks inherent in the surgical act. This survey found that there are many articles dealing with complications after liposuction for aesthetic purposes, and pulmonary fat embolism has a high incidence. Keywords: Lipectomy. Post-operative complications. Fat embolism.

Development:

<u>**Results and discussion:**</u>

Among the case reports of uncommon complications, the following were found: one case of vascular injury with perforation of a large vessel during liposuction(9); two cases of intestinal perforation (9); four articles reporting serious bacterial infections after liposuction (10); one case of herpes zoster; one report of ureteral injury; and three articles on loss of vision associated with liposuction, but in one of the publications the patient already had idiopathic intracranial hypertension, two of these in the last five years (11). Four well-performed experimental studies were selected which dealt with complications in liposuction (5). Three of these studies were carried out on rats of the same Wistar strain and one article used pigs as an animal model. These studies report varying incidences of pulmonary embolism after liposuction, with a higher incidence of pulmonary embolism in rats after liposuction in the studies by El-Ali & Gourlay(8) and Senen et al.(1) than in the study by Franco et al.(12,13).

Pulmonary fat embolism after liposuction can often go undiagnosed, as the clinical presentation can be very variable, ranging from mild dyspnea, tachycardia, elevated temperature and petechiae on the skin to cases of severe respiratory failure, which can lead to death. Its symptoms are unspecific and it is often confused with pulmonary thromboembolism, resulting from deep vein thrombosis (14,15). The exact risk of pulmonary fat embolism is not known, but it is known that death occurs in 15% of diagnosed cases.

A pertinent question, found in Mentz's article (14), is: How many subclinical cases have gone unnoticed and have not been diagnosed and published to date? Grazer & Jong(5) presented a table of articles with a very variable incidence of mortality in liposuction, the highest being 162 per 100,000 cases and the lowest in elective abdominal wall herniorrhaphy, with 3 per 100,000 cases.

Teimourian & Rogers (14) carried out a retrospective study of 75,000 operated cases and reported an incidence of complications > 0.1%, including deep vein thrombosis, pulmonary thromboembolism, fat embolism, skin loss, anesthetic complications, cardiac arrhythmias, organ perforation, bleeding and transfusion-related complications. In this article, 2 patients died as a result of fat embolism and thromboembolism, with an incidence of 2.6 per 100,000. Costa et al.(10) described the case of a Caucasian woman who, after bilateral mastopexy, abdominal liposuction and fat grafting to the buttocks, developed progressive dyspnea and a dry cough on the third day after surgery, with no other symptoms, and was admitted to the intensive care unit. Clinical examination revealed tachypnea, tachycardia, hypoxia on room air, with no changes in lung auscultation; radiography showed minimal bilateral interstitial infiltrates. The patient worsened on the second day of hospital admission, with respiratory acidosis, and was intubated and placed on assisted ventilation. After several tests, acute respiratory failure secondary to fat embolism syndrome was diagnosed. The patient improved on the eighth day of intubation and was extubated and discharged after one month in hospital(16).

Fat embolism in liposuction is a rare condition, but it represents a serious complication of this procedure, with several cases reported. However, the symptoms are unspecific and often underestimated, and the exact risk in liposuction cases has not been established. Fat embolism syndrome is defined as the presence of 2 out of 3 clinical symptoms, including petechiae on the skin, pulmonary discomfort and mental disorders, in the first 48 hours after a trauma. According to Costa et al.(10), these findings are defined by the Gurd and Wilson criteria and are used to help make the diagnosis. According to a publication by Mentz(14), despite the technique used in liposuction, fatty tissues and blood vessels are damaged, causing a flood of fat emboli into the bloodstream. After liposuction, the treated area has residual particles of fat globules and lipids that fall into the circulation. The particles of fat and/or triglycerides that fall into the venous circulation mechanically obstruct the pulmonary circulation or cause a local biochemical inflammatory reaction, situations that cause damage to the endothelium, causing pulmonary spasm, hemorrhages, edema and pulmonary impairment. Emboli that pass through the pulmonary circulation can damage the brain, kidneys, liver and other organs, causing further problems. Fat embolism syndrome shows fat droplets in both lung lavage and urine, which is accompanied by symptoms such as tachycardia, tachypnea, high temperature, hypoxia, thrombocytopenia and neurological disorders. Once a diagnosis is suspected, the treatment to be instituted is clinical support (14). Based on the data collected, Tables 1 to 3 were drawn up (see annexes).

According to other authors consulted (17): Evaldo A. D'Assumpçâo, Luiz Pimentel, Rolf Gemperli, Ricardo Baroudi, the methods of pre-, per- and post-operative prevention of thromboembolic accidents (TEA) routinely used in their liposuction operations are: Pre-operatively, as in any other surgery, perform the classic assessment of the degrees of risk for TEA using the Weinman points system. Do not operate on patients at high risk. I have never taken any preventive medication before, during or after surgery. Perform continuous or intermittent compression of MM.II., early mobilization and elastic stockings.

Careful history-taking, especially regarding the use of medications such as contraceptives, herbal medicines, among others, and personal and family history. In addition, routine blood tests and a thorough clinical examination.

In preoperative prevention, in young patients up to the age of 40, where the liposuction operation is limited to a few areas and a small amount, no special care is taken, with the exception of adequate hydration.

In older patients, or patients with a larger volume to be removed, we use elastic leg stockings, passive movement during surgery and early ambulation.

In the post-operative period, early active and passive physiotherapy, elastic compression and strict hydration are recommended.

Other authors (17) do not use any pharmacological therapy from the pre- to post-operative period, nor do they use elastic containment stockings in the trans-operative period.

They always determine early ambulation, as soon as anesthetic conditions permit.

Once at home, the patient is instructed to move around and rest alternately, depending on the volume and number of regions aspirated.

The same literature reviewed the differential diagnosis between thromboembolism and fat embolism:

However, we can say that the diagnosis of thromboembolism of the lower limbs is made through clinical signs (edema, pain, increased volume, etc.) and ultrasound of the limbs.

Do not combine intracavitary surgeries with abdominoplasties and liposuction, with or without a change of decubitus, in order to avoid risks other than those inherent to the surgeries. Intracavitary surgery (hysterectomy, omentectomy, salpingotripsy, cysts, etc.) and cosmetic abdominoplasties can still be combined in a single operation as long as there are no factors contrary to this indication.

In our humble opinion, we believe that liposuction is more aggressive the greater the number of regions and the volume of fat aspirated. Based on this concept, the occurrence of TEA is directly proportional to megalipos. Worldwide statistics have confirmed this. Always have the criterion of not exceeding 2,500ml of floating fat aspirated in a single operative time(16).

When there are points of adherence of the skin to the aponeurosis, it is clear that there has been a complete "lipectomy" of the subcutaneous tissue, therefore including superficial fascia and connective tissue, and not a true liposuction, which should only aspirate fat cells and preferably from the deep layer. In these cases, it is recommended that you keep it for a year or more and do endermologie-type massage sessions. If possible, liposuction should then be performed on these localized points and, in cases where liposuction was not recommended due to excess skin and pregnancy sequelae, an abdominoplasty.

If it's possible to equalize the denser areas, we perform complementary liposuction. In cases of intense adhesions, the areas are selectively released with a cannula and fatty tissue is interposed. Experience has shown that the results of both the first and second procedures are unsatisfactory, due to the high rate of recurrence of adhesions and the maintenance of asymmetries.

In some cases, careful detachment of the skin flap from the abdominal wall was attempted, with removal of its excess and resection of the excess fatty tissue.

The first option is not to accept the case for treatment, given the limitations on the quality of the result due to the extent of the problems. Referring them to the person who carried out the procedure seems the most logical course of action. It is imperative to clarify the limits and possibilities of the result in advance, as well as whether it will take one or more operative times. The extent of skin laxity, asymmetries in the thickness of the various regions of the post-lipo abdomen and the degree of adherence of the skin to the aponeurosis will determine specific procedures, as summarized below:

1 - New selective liposuction to even out the thickness of the fat pannus, combined with fat injections in the areas of adhesions in one or more operative times.

2 - Liposuction to even out fat thickness combined with a new abdominoplasty. The latter aims to reduce or eliminate any sagging skin.

3 - Follow the procedures in item 2, waiting a minimum of 4 to 6 months before starting fat injections in the areas of adhesions. This last type of procedure involves releasing the adhesions with special stilettos, followed by fat injections.

4 - If fat injections fail, skin resections are indicated along the "lines of force". The scars are less noticeable. We have only had one case where this type of procedure was carried out.

According to Dr. Evaldo A. and at. (17) patients are warned of the possibility of asymmetrical healing. The trochanteric region is also, more rarely, the target of these corrections. The only way to completely avoid such undulations is to only operate on young patients, with small volumes, elastic skin without stretch marks, and tense fat. But this is not the reality that all colleagues have to face. The truth is that it would be very good if everyone were more selective in their liposuction recommendations.

In every surgical procedure, it must be made clear that there is the possibility of future corrections of asymmetries or unsightly scars. From our point of view, this is part of the primary procedure.

We can draw some interesting conclusions. Firstly, we found that the rate of TEAs (thromboembolic accidents), in the vast experience of surgeons who have been dealing with liposuction for a long time, is practically zero. This is in line with many other professionals who also have extensive experience in this field. And we have also confirmed this with our cases. Another curious fact is that none of them - and we too - use preventative medication for such accidents. The general preference is for other approaches, especially moving patients early, which is considered to be more effective. This is borne out by the lack of TIAs in our clinics(18).

With regard to complications from other services, we were struck by Dr. Baroudi's proposal: as far as possible, not to operate on such cases, but to return them to the original surgeon. Such behavior may seem unsympathetic, but it seems to us to be right. Correction attempts, even if they give satisfactory results, almost always fall far short of what we could have given the patient in a primary procedure. For this very reason, there will almost always not be complete fulfillment for the person making the correction, and there may also be dissatisfaction on the part of the patient, if they had higher expectations of our work. On the other hand, if he is satisfied, he will certainly present the result to his friends, making it out to be the surgeon's alone, almost never referring to the author of the first procedure. The precarious result will certainly look as if it were the ordinary result of someone who only undertook an attempt at correction.

Finally, the question of charging fees for correcting the work itself takes a common path: everyone considers the touch-ups to be part of the initial treatment and doesn't charge anything for them. This attitude seems somewhat complex to us, as not being paid for the correction opens the way for the surgeon to be charged for hospital costs as well. If he doesn't work in his own clinic, he will certainly face significant costs. On the other hand, a charge may not be well accepted by the patient and could lead to conflicts that end up in legal proceedings. Sometimes a bad deal is better than a good fight.

We believe that, in these circumstances, a well-managed doctor-patient relationship is vital for the surgeon. If there has been no error, it will be essential to show this calmly to the patient, even offering not to charge a fee, but making it clear that the hospital expenses will be borne by the patient. However, if there has been a medical error, no matter how minor, it would be wise not to create any friction by trying to solve the patient's problem without the patient having to pay anything. In this way, you will avoid a relationship breakdown that will only harm the surgeon.

For all these reasons, it is essential to have a well-drafted "Informed Consent", always signed by the patient and a witness, after thorough explanations, without omitting any possible complications for fear of losing the patient.

According to other authors (14,18) infection can be a consequence of techniques combined with lipectomy, the formation of hematomas and seromas can become sources of infection, hence the importance of meticulous hemostasis and seroma drainage. In addition, adopting aseptic techniques throughout the procedure is essential. The use of prophylactic antibiotics is controversial.

Tumescent liposuction produces deep hemostasis. The ideal ratio of liquid infused into the subcutaneous space to liquid aspirated is controversial, and excessive infiltration should be avoided.

As with any surgical procedure, there are risks which must always be explained to the candidate for this type of procedure. among others, the following complications are listed:

. Unfavorable scars;

• Bleeding (hematoma);

• Accumulation of fluid (seroma);

• Anesthetic risks;

• Poor healing;

• Skin necrosis;

• Numbness or other changes in skin sensitivity;

• Asymmetry;

• Skin depigmentation and/or prolonged swelling;

• Burn caused by ultrasound - ultrasound-assisted liposuction technique;

• Damage to deeper structures such as nerves, blood vessels, muscles and lungs;

• Pain that can last;

• Deep vein thrombosis, cardiac and pulmonary complications;

• Suture threads can spontaneously emerge in the skin, becoming visible or causing irritation that requires removal;

• Possibility of a new surgical procedure.

The available literature highlights the most frequent minor complications:

• Contour irregularities, better defined as a sequel rather than a real complication, can occur in any treated area. According to some articles, it has been reported that ultrasound-assisted liposuction (UAOL) presents fewer problems of this type which can be avoided by performing the procedure in an orderly manner (5). - Hypoesthesia of the skin located in the liposuction area is a normal and expected sequence of liposuction. The post-operative theoretical synthesis of anti-inflammatory and desensitizing genes. Howard found a direct relationship between the amplitude of ultrasound energy and the degree of nerve damage in a study carried out on rats in 1998 (5).

• Theoretically, all treated areas are swollen, so compression garments should be worn during the post-operative period to reduce this complication (6).

• Ecchymosis will be inevitable in response to the injury to small vessels, which in most cases will resolve spontaneously; however, hemosiderin staining can be permanent without any treatment for it (2,5,6). - Post-operative bleeding can be frequent, which can be avoided by adequate tissue infiltration with epinephrine solutions which, due to their vasoconstrictive effect, reduce bleeding from small vascular lesions. Therefore, check the extracted material carefully. If ultrasound is used, it should only be used in infiltrated areas. The use of worn titanium cannulas has also been associated with tissue trauma and potential bleeding (5).

• The appearance of seromas has been seen more frequently with the use of ultrasound. They are more frequent when large amounts of fat are removed or when the procedure is combined with open surgery. Their frequency can be reduced by limiting the time of exposure to ultrasound and placing post-operative drainage, (7, 8).

• Fortunately, infection is not a common complication in liposuction and can be prevented with proper washing and sterilization of the equipment, as well as the use of adequate asepsis and antisepsis during the procedure itself. The germ most often involved is Staphylococcus aureus. Prophylactic antibiotics such as first-generation cephalosporins are commonly used (5).

• Cases of necrotizing fasciitis have also been reported, with the most frequent microorganisms being anaerobes and beta hemolytic streptococci. Treatment includes a combination of broad-spectrum antibiotics, aggressive debridement and the administration of hyperbaric oxygen (5).

Skin necrosis resulting from a bascular or thermal injury can be completely avoided if the technique is performed correctly and respecting the anatomy. Thermal subcutaneous space injury is one of the only avoidable risks of ultrasound-assisted liposuction, considering its two main rules: applying ultrasound only to the infiltrated tissue and always keeping the cannula moving (15,18).

Due to the small diameter and length of the cannulas and the blind nature of the procedure, there is a risk of directing the cannula into unwanted tissue planes, resulting in the perforation of a viscera. Patients at high risk of intestinal perforation are considered to be those with abdominal wall hernia; a history of abdominal surgery, including laparoscopy, due to pneumoperitoneum, so the physical examination should emphasize looking for abdominal scars and any hernia that alerts the surgeon to a risk of perforation. Tomography and ultrasound have also been used in patients in whom the physical examination is doubtful, as is the case with obese patients (18).

Deep vein thrombosis

Pulmonary embolism is a common disease in our hospital environment and a frequent cause of death. The incidence of deep vein thrombosis is approximately 0.1 to 0.8% in patients without prophylaxis. Although there is little information on this complication in cosmetic surgery patients, the risk seems to be low (15,18,19,20).

It is a fact that untreated pulmonary embolism should be considered a disease state with relatively high mortality if not properly diagnosed.

Clinical manifestations are variable and unspecific and may or may not show signs or symptoms, even when there is extensive deep thrombosis. Symptoms can be pain or tightness in the leg, with or without inflammation, pain on passive heel dorsiflexion, Homan's sign and when pulmonary embolism occurs there can be pleuritic pain, dyspnea, hemoptysis, tachycardia, tachypnea, altered mental state or sudden respiratory decompensation in the postoperative period (15,21).

Risk factors

The most important step in diagnosing pulmonary thromboembolism is clinical suspicion.

It is essential to first consider the risk factors, among which the important antecedents are:

Pathological context:

I.Various genetic and acquired defects predispose patients to developing bleeding coagulation disorders, such as dysphrenogenemia and abnormalities of factors VIII, IX and X

2   Hypercoagulable states including abnormal prothrombin, normal or absent antithrombin III, abnormal protein C O S, abnormal platelets and antiphospholipid syndrome.

3   . Patients with a previous history of pulmonary embolism, chronic venous insufficiency.

4 Obesity

5   Surgical or non-surgical trauma

5.1   severe systemic infection

7 Controversy

8   Central nervous system disease or peripheral paralysis of the lower limbs

9   Homocysteinemia

10. Radiotherapy, especially for pelvic neoplasms

11. Women taking oral contraceptives or hormone replacement have a higher risk.

12. Pregnancy

13. Heart disease

14. Diseases involving prolonged immobilization

A history of thrombotic events or hypercoagulable states is important in the family history. These factors are further modified by the patient's general care, duration and type of anesthesia, perioperative immobilization, degree of dehydration and presence of sepsis. Therefore, the individual risk is determined by the type of surgery and the accumulation of predisposing factors.

The diagnosis will therefore be the result of the sum of risk factors, signs and symptoms, EKG, chest X-ray, ventilation/perfusion test, however, the most accurate test to confirm the diagnosis is pulmonary arteriography.

Prophylaxis and management

In October 1998, the American Society of Plastic and Reconstructive Surgery created the "forced force" in pulmonary thromboembolism, which consists of several recommendations, taking into account the clinical history, physical examination and appropriate laboratory tests, the risk of deep vein thrombosis is classified as low, moderate and high, which determines prophylactic treatment (21) (Table 1).

The most common prophylactic measures are:

1. Early ambulance: should be started before 24 hours gradually.

2. Graduated compression stockings: have been observed to increase the rate of venous blood flow, although there is no conclusive evidence that they prevent or reduce the incidence of pulmonary embolism.

3. Intermittent compression of the lower limbs: increases deep venous blood flow and promotes fibrinolytic activity.

4. Oral anticoagulants: the use of aspirin is not recommended as prophylaxis. In high-risk patients, in very select cases, perioperative warfarin with an INR of 2 to 3 can be used.

5. Heparin: usually administered in low doses of 5000U. subcutaneously 2 hours before surgery and post-operatively every 8 or 12 hours, depending on the risk.

6. Low molecular weight heparins (LMWH): their best effectiveness in preventing thrombosis has been demonstrated. They have a good preventive effect when administered in the first 24 hours after surgery. In our setting, enoxiparin is recommended at 20 mg subcutaneously/day with moderate risk and 20 mg every 12 hours with high risk and nadroparin at 40 U/kg 2 hours before surgery and once a day for three days (19,20,21).

Fat thrombolism is another complication of liposuction. The available statistics are associated with long bone fractures (18,19), but those associated with liposuction are not described.

By assimilation, the same pathophysiology that occurs in polytrauma with fracture of the long bones (18) has been suggested, although in liposuction it is not clear if it is the same mechanism. It is thought to be due to neutral fat from the affected area being embolized into the pulmonary circulation where it is hydrolyzed by lipase present in the pneumocytes into free fatty acids which are chemically harmful to the lung parenchyma, leading to acute respiratory distress syndrome.

Symptoms occur during the first 24 hours in 60% of cases, within 48 hours in 85% and rarely after 72 hours (15) and are characterized by tachycardia, tachypnea, fever, hypoxemia, mental disorientation, lethargy and irritability. Petechial hemorrhages are a classic manifestation and occur in 50% of patients. There is also a rash in the axillary folds, flanks, buccal mucosa, conjunctiva and retinal infarcts. Ocular manifestations are characteristic, but transient, such as eyelid edema, white spots or retinal hemorrhages. Laboratory studies show an increase in serum lipase, anemia, thrombocytopenia and hypocalcemia, as well as hypocholesterolemia and an increase in free fatty acids. Fat globules can be found in urine and sputum. The chest X-ray shows the image of snow, characteristic of pulmonary edema. These findings usually occur in the first 24 to 72 hours (15).

In patients with a history of trauma and usually with long bone fractures, methylprednisolone is used as prophylaxis at a dose of 30 mg/kg, which is repeated at 4 hours (19). According to the recommendation of the American Society of Plastic and Reconstructive Surgery with its team in the evaluation of liposuction (15), once the diagnosis of fat embolism is suspected, high doses of corticosteroids should be started. The recommended dose of methylprednisolone is 15 to 30 mg/kg in a 20-minute infusion, continuing every 6 hours for a total of 48 hours. This is associated with all oxygen measures, intubation, PEEP and mechanical ventilation according to each case.

Despite these reports, there are still many issues regarding the pathophysiology and diagnosis of fat embolism in liposuction patients. It is possible, given the nature of the procedure, to find fat-free blood cells in the blood or urine without the syndrome occurring.

Medicines and liposuction

Over time, various contributions have been made to improve the liposuction technique, including the introduction of the blunt cannula and anterior infiltration, Illouz, until reaching the tumescent technique, introduced by Klein in 1987. It has been shown to be a safe procedure, but there must be important considerations regarding its application.

Lidocaine

In 1995, this drug began to be used in patients undergoing large-volume liposuction, increasing the rate of complications, apparently due to overdose of lidocaine with overhydration (20). Lidocaine is the local anesthetic of choice due to its lower toxicity compared to bupivacaine or other local anesthetics. The maximum dose recommended by the manufacturer is 7 mg / kg, without exceeding a total dose of 500 mg (22,23,24).

The toxic effects observed with its administration depend on the serum levels reached, as follows:

3-6 ug / ml Subjective effects

5-9 ug / ml Objective toxicity *

8-12 ug / ml Convulsions, cardiac depression

12 ug / ml Coma

20 ug / ml Respiratory arrest

26 ug / ml Cardiac arrest.

- Visual and auditory alterations, restlessness, numbness of the tongue and muscle fasciculations (22, 25).

The rate of absorption of lidocaine will depend on its concentration, the vascularity of the injection site, the concomitant use of the vasoconstrictor and the rate of infiltration.

The maximum plasma concentration occurs around 90 minutes after subcutaneous infiltration. Diluting lidocaine in a solution containing epinephrine decreases its absorption rate and toxicity (23).

Several studies have shown that it is safe to infiltrate 35-55 mg/kg of lidocaine when it is accompanied by epinephrine and injected into the subcutaneous fat, with a low infiltration rate and segmental infiltration, because in this way its absorption is much slower, reducing the maximum plasma levels (26,27,28).

It is recommended to calculate the maximum dose according to the patient's composition (13):

- 45 mg / kg in thin patients

- 55 mg / kg in the average patient

- 60 mg / kg in overweight patients

Another group of patients in whom the calculated dose should be lowered is elderly and male patients in whom the applied dose should be reduced by 20-30%.

Lidocaine serum peaks after infusion of the solution at 12-24 hours. Doses higher than those recommended by the manufacturer can be used, since when lidocaine is used diluted under the conditions mentioned above, its systemic absorption takes 18 to 36 hours (2), reaching maximum non-toxic serum levels.

In some special cases, care should be taken with the calculated dose. This is the case for patients who are taking drugs that inhibit or compete with cytochrome P4503A4, where the enzyme responsible for its metabolism is found (3), for example, if they are taking new generation antidepressants, serotonin reuptake inhibitors, the calculated dose should be reduced by 30 to 40%.

Other drugs that should be treated are benzodiazepines, imidazoles, macrolides, anticonvulsants, propofol, propranolol and thyroxine (13).

It is suggested that, in the case of liposuction under general anesthesia, lidocaine should not be included in the infiltrate, as its use is not necessary during the procedure and, in one study, it was reported that its post-operative effect is very low or non-existent (15).

Some final recommendations to avoid overdosing with lidocaine include:

1 Know the correct dose for each patient

2 Specify this dose in terms of milligrams.

3 Use only 1% lidocaine.

4 Supervising the preparation of the infiltrate.

5 Keep the empty bottles until the end.

6 . Avoid the use of benzodiazepines. in the postoperative period (14).

Adrenaline

It is a direct sympathetic agonist drug that is used for its vasoconstrictive effect on arterioles and precapillary sphincters. It is unquestionable that its addition to infiltrated solutions has significantly reduced blood loss (23).

The side effects associated with its administration are: fear of anxiety, tension, headache, tremor, weakness, palpitations, tachycardia and cardiac arrhythmias. There are no studies on its dosage in liposuction.

Appetite suppressants

In the pharmacological context, it is very important to detect various drugs that patients sometimes don't know about or hide from the attending doctor.

It should be borne in mind that many of the patients seeking liposuction are overweight patients who have tried various methods to lose weight, sometimes including appetite suppressant drugs.

They are mainly sympathomimetic amines that act by modulating the release and reuptake of serotonin and norepinephrine. Among the most widely used is phenylpropanolamine, which is also present in antifungals and antitussives.

Their association with cerebral events such as ischemia, hemorrhage and vasculitis is well documented in the literature (29,30).

Fluid, electrolyte and blood replacement.

The surgeon must have a complete knowledge of electrolyte requirements and the possibility of transfusion in the patient undergoing liposuction, as important post-operative changes occur in this procedure.

In 1986, Hetter compared liposuction to a burn or hematoma. The soft tissue compartment, which has been depleted of fat with liposuction, sequesters large quantities of fluids, electrolytes, albumin and blood. This sequestration of fluid and blood is mainly evidenced by the edema and bruising that the patient presents post-operatively at the level of the liposuction areas (1).

In 1988, Dr. Hetter himself showed that the hematocrit drops by 1% for every 88cc of fat aspirated 48 hours after liposuction. By administering a 1:400,000 solution of epinephrine to a 0.25% solution of lidocaine, the hematocyst fell by 1% for every 136 cc of fat aspirated within 48 hours of the procedure (31). This rule predicts that if lidocaine with epinephrine is infiltrated in an amount of 15 to 30 cc per 100 cm2 of area to be treated, the hematocrit drops by 1% for every 150 cc of aspirate(32,33).

This rule only applies if the aspirate is not excessively bloody. According to this rule, in a liposuction of 1500 cc of aspirate, the hematocrit decreases by 10%. This rule does not differentiate between internal and external blood loss. Internal blood loss is secondary to trauma within the liposuction tissues and represents intravascular blood loss into the extracellular space. External blood loss accompanies the aspirate and is represented by the volume of blood recovered in the reservoir bottle at the end of the procedure.(32)

Several attempts have been made to estimate external blood loss by determining the lipocrit, which represents the percentage of blood in a fat aspirate. Grazer (1983) mentioned an estimate of between 10-15% (33), Courtiss (1984) estimated 33% (38) and Pitman (1991) estimated 44% (34).

Using a biochemical measurement method, Goodpasture and Bunkis (1986) found variations of between 8 and 54% in the blood/fat gain ratio. The investigations mentioned varied in wet and dry techniques, the size of the cannulas used, the time taken to complete the aspiration and the method of determining lipocrit (35).

In general terms, lipocrit can be determined in two ways:

1. Obtaining the patient's preoperative hemoglobin and measuring the hemoglobin in the aspirate, divide the total amount of Hb aspirated between the preoperative Hb concentration (36).

2. Allow the aspirate to separate by gravitation for two hours. Take two

infranatant samples to determine hemoglobin and mean. The total amount of hemoglobin in the infranatant is determined by multiplying the hemoglobin by the volume of the infranatant. The total amount of blood lost in the infranatant is calculated by dividing the total amount of hemoglobin by the hemoglobin concentration in a preoperative blood sample.

However, the estimate of external blood loss is not as relevant as the rule of 150, which estimates total blood loss with any technique used.

Pitman (8) proposes calculating total blood loss based on preoperative hematocrit, postoperative hematocrit, estimated blood volume and patient weight:

Hcto preop-Hcto POP (%) X estimated blood volume x weight Hcto preop.

The total blood volume in adults is 65 cc / kg in women and 70 cc / kg in men.

Healthy young adult patients can easily tolerate a blood volume loss of 25% without transfusion. Acute losses of 40% of blood volume are clinically associated with significant hypotension, even when hydroterrolyte replacement is performed. In general terms, it is accepted that an extraction of 1750 cc of fat aspirate predicts the need for autotransfusion in healthy adults.

To pre-operatively estimate the need for autotransfusion, Hetter uses the analogy of liposuction with a burn, giving an important predictive value to the percentage of body surface area. According to this rule, if the surface area of the body to be operated on exceeds 15%, hemodynamic instability will occur and the need for autotransfusion can be anticipated (32,36).

The percentage estimate depending on the area is determined as 4 to 8% in the abdomen, 2 to 4% in the flanks, 6 to 12% in the lateral thigh region and 2 to 4% in the mid-thigh region.

It should be remembered that there are various forms of subcutaneous infiltration of the solution (Table 2).

Pitman and Holzer (1991) showed that the average water replacement has a linear relationship with the volume of fat aspirated and defined guidelines for electrolyte replacement based on the volume of fat aspirated (39). The total volume of crystalloids administered should be double the volume of fat aspirated, of which 50% is administered intraoperatively and 50% postoperatively. However, it should be borne in mind that Pitamn and Molzer use a wet technique (35,36).

Rohrich, Beran and Fodor (1997) reviewed the literature on water substitution according to the technique used (37, 38,39), and made the following recommendations:

Dry technique

Less than 1500 ml aspirated: Replace 2: 1 intravenous / aspirated liquid 1,500 ml - 3000 ml aspirated: 1 unit of autologous blood and 2: 1 intravenous / aspirated liquid. Greater than 3000 ml aspirated: 2 units of autologous blood and 2: 1 intravenous / aspirated liquid.

Wet technique

Less than 2,500 ml of aspirate: 1:1 intravenous fluid/ aspirate intraoperatively and 1:1 intravenous fluid/ aspirate postoperatively.

Greater than 2,500 ml of aspirate: intravenous fluid 1:1 aspirated / aspirated intraoperatively; 1:1 intravenous fluid aspirated / aspirated POP + 1-2 U blood if Hct <30.

Super-wet technique

<3000 ml of aspirate: <1: 1 intravenous fluid aspirate / aspirate, early oral initiation> 3000 ml of aspirate: 1: 1 intravenous fluid aspirate / aspirate, early oral initiation, monitoring of urine production.

Tumescent technique

<3000 ml of aspirate: <1: 1 aspirate / intravenous liquid aspirate and early oral initiation. > 3000 ml of aspirate: 1: 1 aspirate / intravenous liquid, early oral initiation.

With regard to autotransfusion, it is considered that the units should be taken at least one week in advance, in order to allow for adequate compensatory erythrocytosis. Packed red blood cells can remain in the blood bank for up to 6 weeks. Iron supplementation should be started at the time of blood drawing and continued for up to 6 weeks after surgery(40,41).

If more than one unit of autotransfusion blood is needed, it should be taken at one-week intervals. Hetter recommends whole blood whenever possible, because it provides replacement albumin and red blood cells and possibly avoids pulmonary complications after surgery. The transfusion should be done at the end of the procedure or during recovery (42,43).

When autotransfusion must be performed, adequate diuresis monitoring must be carried out during and after surgery, and the patient must remain hospitalized with intravenous fluids of between 75 and 125 cc per hour.

Water balance

There is the same risk of water imbalance in conventional liposuction as in ultrasound-assisted liposuction.

With the introduction of the tumescent technique, the prevention of water imbalance focused especially on the possibility of water overload, rather than hypovolemia. This technique represents a ratio of infiltrated volume to aspirated volume of 3:1.

Gilliland et al. present pulmonary edema as a potential complication of liposuction. They recommend a complete clinical history to rule out cardiovascular, pulmonary, renal or hepatic pathology; permanent communication with the anesthesiologist and the use of Ringer's lactate rather than saline in order to reduce the sodium load. Urine output should be maintained at 1 cc / kg / hour during the procedure (44,45,46).

Commons and Halprin recommend the residual volume theory to measure the amount of residual fluid in the patient after large volumes of liposuction. This theory takes into account the amount of solution remaining in the subcutaneous tissue, the intravenous fluids administered during the procedure, the amount of solution aspirated and the outflow of urine. The volume of fat aspirated is not included in the equation.

They found that patients with a residual volume of wet solution of less than 70 cc / Kg correlated with stable vital signs, with no evidence of water overload. Diuretics should be used in patients with a residual volume of more than 70 cc / Kg, (49) (Volume of tumescent solution + Volume of intravenous fluids) - (Volume of tumescent solution aspirated + Urinary expenditure + Estimated deduction in the first hour of recovery) = Volume of residual water.

Pulmonary edema

There are two types of pulmonary edema: cardiogenic pulmonary edema or high pulmonary pressure, which occurs when there is circulatory overload or left heart failure, which produces an excess of pulmonary capillary hydrostatic pressure over plasma oncotic pressure, favoring the transudation of fluid into the alveolus. Non-cardiogenic pulmonary edema results from damage to the alveolar membrane, allowing fluid to pass into the alveolus (47). A typical example of this condition is the lung damage seen in adult respiratory distress syndrome.

In the specific case of pulmonary edema as a complication of liposuction, cardiogenic edema, excessive accumulation of water in the interstitial and alveolar spaces of the lung, alters the hydrological control factors in the lung. These factors are capillary and tissue pressure, interstitial and plasma oncotic pressures, capillary permeability and lymph flow. Capillary and tissue pressures are low, but with the influence of oncotic pressure, since the pulmonary capillaries easily allow the filtration of proteins, there is always significant filtration which is compensated for by the lymph flow.

A rapid and significant increase in plasma volume results in a rise in central venous pressure and in pulmonary arterial volume and pressure. The normal lung has a great capacity to regulate these changes, especially by recruiting lung areas that normally lack volume and high blood flow.

Patients who start with an increase in blood volume and are administered large volumes of water are unable to compensate with lymph flow and the water expands first into the interstitial space and then into the alveolar space. In these situations, an excessive dilution of plasma proteins and the consequent decrease in oncotic pressure can facilitate the filtration of water into the interstitium. The risk of pulmonary edema is determined by the pre-existing clinical condition and the speed and volume of water administered (47,48).

Once the risk of water overload has been established, it is important to recognize the first signs of pulmonary edema. The use of a pulse oximeter is very helpful because it identifies hypoxemia and interstitial pulmonary edema early on.

The formation of interstitial edema decreases lung compliance and increases the work of breathing, causing dyspnea, tachypnea and mild hypoxemia. Bronchial narrowing due to edema produces expiratory wheezing and cardiac asthma. If the process progresses, alveolar flooding occurs, exacerbating pulmonary dysfunction and worsening hypoxemia. Other signs associated with pulmonary edema are hypertension, tachycardia and diaphoresis.

In the early stages, interstitial edema can be seen on the chest X-ray by the presence of septal lines, peribronchial and perivascular rings and accentuation of the interlobar fissure. Cephalization of the pulmonary vasculature and opacification of the hilae are characteristic findings. Progression to alveolar flooding produces a diffuse bilateral infiltrate.

During the procedure, it is important to minimize the administration of intravenous fluids (47). If water retention is suspected immediately after surgery, diuretics should be administered, furosemide at a dose of 20-40 mg IV every 6 hours.

Pulmonary edema requires urgent attention. Cardiogenic pulmonary edema resolves quickly after the volume overload is corrected. In most surgical patients, pulmonary artery catheterization is necessary to distinguish between cardiogenic and non-cardiogenic pulmonary edema. The wedge pressure, which reflects the end-diastolic pressure in the left ventricle, is between 20 and 25 mm Hg, cardiac output is low and systemic vascular resistance is high in cardiogenic pulmonary edema. A normal wedge pressure of 1015 mm Hg and a normal or high cardiac output suggests low pressure pulmonary edema or adult respiratory distress syndrome(49).

Immediate measures include sitting the patient on their right side to improve lung compliance, reduce the effort of breathing and reduce cardiac preload.

Hypoxemia is treated with 100% oxygen administration and, if it doesn't respond, ventilatory support should be established. Endotracheal intubation and positive pressure ventilation can decrease interstitial water, as it increases lymphatic flow and maintains high alveolar pressures, minimizing the possibility of alveolar flooding.

The administration of low doses of dopamine, 2-5 micrograms/kg/min, increases renal flow and promotes diuresis. In situations where diuresis is inadequate, hemofiltration is highly effective in rapidly reducing intravascular volume.

Reducing afterload with sodium nitroprusside is useful in patients with high systemic vascular resistance (50).

It is important to determine previous reactions to local anesthetics, tachycardia with infiltrations for previous procedures, the patient's current nutritional status and their weight and height.

Special care should be taken with the following patients:

- hypertensive, and patients with cardiovascular disease, a history suggestive of pheochromocytoma, hyperthyroidism, carcinoid tumor, those taking pseudoephedrine, influenza and nutritional supplements with a product similar to ephedrine; all of these because of their greater susceptibility to exogenous catecholamines.

- diabetics, for the increased risk of infection and scarring, especially when they are not well controlled, in addition to reducing the load - tolerance liquids according to the commitment having target organ.

- Epilepsy and other seizure syndromes, patients who would be difficult to determine whether they are convulsing during the procedure due to the underlying disease or lidocaine neurotoxicity.

- Patients with hepatitis will have an impaired liver metabolism. Those with HIV will have an unacceptably increased risk of infection, as well as biosafety problems.

- With regard to patients who are receiving previous treatment with anticoagulants, it is important to bear in mind that prophylactic anticoagulation should be suspended 12-24 hours before the procedure and aspirin should be discontinued 10 days beforehand.

- Non-steroidal anti-inflammatory drugs should be discontinued three days beforehand. It's important to take special care of those who take vitamin E chronically. They are statistically more likely to bleed. MAO inhibitors and zertraline: arrhythmogenic effect, cimetidine, slows down the metabolism of lidocaine, and in pure vegetarians there is an increase in healing time.

In addition to the general recommendations for preoperative assessment and the request for pre-surgical tests by the anesthesia service, these patients will be asked for: complete blood count, PT, PTT, hemoclasification with typing and antibody screening and patients with clinical suspicion of malnutrition, total proteins and albumin (51,52).

It is important to write down in the medical history the permitted doses of lidocaine for the patient according to their weight and to sign the consent form, as proof that the procedure is accepted and known.

Anesthesia

Small area or volume liposuction procedures should preferably be performed with local anesthesia, true tumescent liposuction plus monitored anesthetic care (CAM). Some procedures can be performed adequately and safely with regional epidural anesthesia, depending on the acceptance of the patient, surgeon and surgical time.

In other procedures where general anesthesia is used, inhalation anesthesia, due to its pharmacological characteristics, is very suitable and will be contraindicated in patients with sensitivity to any inhaled anesthetic and in those with risk factors or a history of malignant hyperthermia(26).

Isoflurane, due to its low metabolism and non-interaction with catecholamines, has a very favorable profile. Sevofluorane remains a good choice, without forgetting, at any time, its high percentage of metabolism and interaction with the CO_2 absorber, which can be relevant in procedures lasting longer than four hours.

Halothane sensitizes the myocardium to catecholamines, so it should not be used in procedures where infiltrations with these will be used. Defluorine favors the release of catecholamines at a systemic level and should therefore not be used either.

Hypnotic agents such as propofol and sodium thiopental are suitable for induction. Propofol, due to its half-life and metabolism, can be used as an infusion as the hypnotic component of a balanced anesthetic. In anesthetic induction, any of the new opioids can be used. Especially those with short half-lives, such as remifentanil and alfentanil. Remifentanil, due to its plasma metabolism and ultra-short half-life, is a good option for maintaining balanced anesthesia.

The use of benzodiazepines will be avoided as much as possible due to their sedative and hypnotic characteristics and their pharmacological interaction at the level of cytochrome P 450 with local anesthetics. If co-interaction is necessary, the alternative is midazolam.

In general terms, the use of muscle relaxants is not routinely necessary in this type of surgery. If necessary, those with a short and intermediate half-life will be chosen. These will be reinforced by high doses of local anesthetics(53).

It is always recommended in this type of surgery, under general anesthesia:

- Monitoring

- EKG Continuous

- Non-invasive blood pressure

- Pulse oximetry

- Capnography

- Esophageal stent

- Bladder leakage before the procedure

- Bladder catheter in major surgeries or for more than 3 hours

- Deep venous access and collection of hemoglobin and hematocrit - Solutions.

The solutions should be prepared on the same day for use and should be labeled in mg/l of solution for anesthesia and epinephrine. Lidocaine should always be used to avoid errors. It is preferred to use normal saline (0.9%) as a solvent. The use of bell lactate is not recommended due to the appearance of transient lactoacidosis. (27)

With regard to the use of lidocaine, other authors (28,53) have stated that the limit dose is 45 to 50 mg / kg, depending on the amount of adipose tissue the patient has, with a higher admissible dose for high fat content. As for epinephrine, there is no report of a maximum admissible dose, but we do have data on average infiltrations of 4-6 mg. The major limitation will be the patient's heart rate, where if heart rates exceed 120 beats x min, it is recommended to suspend infiltration and apply clonidine or IV B-blockers. The infiltrations should be carried out sequentially. When you are going to do liposuction of several areas, for example: abdomen and hips, you should first infiltrate and suction the abdomen and then infiltrate and suction each of the hips.

Pre-medication with clonidine 0.075 mg, in addition to sedating the patient and reducing the need for anesthetic agents, avoids the potential risk of tachycardia secondary to epinephrine absorption.

The adverse effects of lidocaine can be summarized as follows:

With doses between 50 and 55 mg / kg, nausea and vomiting can occur during the first 12 hours after surgery. With doses above 55 mg / kg of lidocaine, tachycardia is the main cause. There may be lethargy and sedation, so sedatives are not recommended in the first 24 hours after surgery. In patients taking non-selective B blockers, hypertensive crises have been described.

Management of intravenous fluids (45,51).

For an average patient weighing 60 kg:

1. 100 cc for each hour of fasting (4 cc for the first 10 kilos, 2 cc for the second 10 kilos, 1 cc for each additional kilo).

2. 520 cc of crystalloids for each hour of surgery (100 cc of basal maintenance plus 7 cc per kilo per type of surgery)

3. Bleeding will be replaced with 4:1 crystalloids, 2:1 colloids Haemacel and Gelafundin 2:1 and Gelinfundol 5% 1:1 or blood 1:1. Once you have reached the permitted bleeding before transfusion. It is important to bear in mind that any calculation or estimate before surgery at any time replaces the clinical assessment of the anesthesiologist, the ultimate determinant of the need for fluids and the type of fluids.

Risk factors

- Multiple surgeries in the same intervention

- Large aspirated volume Greater than 5 liters

- Toxic doses of local anesthetics

- Volumes of excess intravenous liquid plus tumescent infiltrate.

- Drug interaction: the metabolism of sedatives decreases with high concentrations of lidocaine.

Mortality

From 1993 to the present day, 130 deaths have been reported in the United States. In Florida there have been 34 cases since 1986 and 13 from 1997 to date. The global mortality incidence has been estimated at 2 per 100,000; however, in recently published reports, it is estimated at approximately 1 in 5200 cases. The main causes of mortality are:

-Hemorrhage and shock.

-Myocardial infarction.

-Pulmonary embolism.

-Drug interaction.

-Infection

- Fasciitis.

Liposuction techniques:(Fig.1,2,3)

In the literature reviewed, we found various techniques for this procedure (45).

Liposculpture

Liposculpture is one of the most popular techniques among women. Some call it a "hole-filling operation", because part of the fat removed is injected into areas that need filling, such as the buttocks, cellulite holes and furrows in the face. There is no risk of rejection, as the fat applied is the client's own.

In the post-operative period, there may be swelling, which requires rest, the use of an elastic waistband and lymphatic drainage sessions. Swelling and blemishes disappear within 21 days in most cases. The results of liposculpture appear 6 months after the operation, but by the fourth month, 80% of the result has already been achieved.

Minilipo:

Minilipo is also known as Lipo Light. It can only be done on areas with a low fat content. Hospitalization is not necessary and the client's routine can be resumed the next day, in some cases. Swelling is common up to five days after the operation, which is why lymphatic drainage sessions are very important.

Hydrolipo:

This technique is best suited to the knees and culottes. Hydrolipo is done with a liquid (Ringer's lactate with lidocaine and adrenaline) that is infiltrated into the area in order to fill up the fatty tissue. It is a less painful procedure, but as it is carried out on various parts of the body, it often requires more than one session, which results in a higher cost.

In the post-operative period, it is necessary to wear an elastic girdle for 4 weeks and to have lymphatic drainage sessions to avoid swelling. The results are excellent, the abdomen is reduced by about 6 cm and the buttocks by 8 cm.

Vibro liposuction:

Vibro-liposuction is an innovative procedure. It consists of the introduction of vibrating mechanisms into the suction cannulas, because once they penetrate the fatty tissue, there is less trauma. Other advantages of this procedure are that there is less bleeding and pain in the post-operative period and recovery is much quicker. In the post-operative period, the use of an elastic band and lymphatic drainage sessions are recommended.

Beverly Hills Lipo:

Requested by big personalities to eliminate small amounts of localized fat, Beverly Hills Lipo arrived in Brazil recently and is already a sensation among women. Much like regular lipo, with the difference that it is done with a much smaller cannula, Beverly Hills Lipo offers a smooth post-operative period and a shorter and more efficient recovery time.

Without leaving any cuts, it doesn't even require a heavy anesthetic, and can be done simply by applying xylocaine and saline solution (local anesthetic).

Laser Lipo:

Attached to the fat aspiration cannulas is a laser-operated device that melts the fat layer, killing the fat cells. However, if the aspiration is not complete, the cells, even if dead, remain in the client's body, which can lead to a lack of regularity on the surface of the skin. The post-operative period should be accompanied by lymphatic drainage sessions and the use of an elastic waistband.

In addition to these techniques, we also have Abdominoplasty, which removes excess skin concentrated in the abdomen, harmonizes proportions, shapes the body, leaves the abdomen looking toned (healed), as well as reducing stretch marks when located in the navel area.

Among the technologies currently available, laser liposuction, better known as lipolaser, is one that has shown the best results, especially in the post-operative period.

According to plastic surgeon Rogério Matoso, lipolaser scars the patient less and facilitates the cauterization process, avoiding major blood loss during the procedure. This allows for better retraction of the skin in the operated area, speeding up the recovery process. "Lipolaser allows us to release patients to their activities more quickly, comfortably and safely. In these cases, the return usually takes around three to four days, while with conventional liposuction, the time off usually lasts between seven and ten days."

This shortening of the post-operative period is due to the way the technique works. In conventional liposuction, the excess fat is sucked out through the device's cannulas. In lipolaser, the fat is first dissolved by the action of the laser and then absorbed by a special cannula connected to the device. This process makes the removal a little less aggressive (Fig. 4A, 4B).

Post-operative care

However, like the other techniques, lipolaser is an invasive procedure that should be carried out in a hospital environment, with adequate infrastructure and security, and by a trained plastic surgeon with experience and mastery of the technology. Likewise, it should not be recommended to patients who are very overweight and want to lose weight. "Liposuction is a surgical procedure to remove so-called 'localized fat'. Its aim is to improve the contour of the body, acting on specific areas such as the abdomen, flanks, waist, thighs etc.", comments Matoso.

The fact that it promotes a faster recovery doesn't mean that lipolaser rules out the post-operative period. On the contrary, the operated patient must take the same care as with other techniques, using a modeling belt, taking the prescribed medication, resting, performing lymphatic drainage, among others.

Various instruments and cannulas have been introduced for liposuction. The tumescent technique, ultrasonic lipo, or laser, are aids to more advanced and safer liposuction, but they do not avoid the risk of aesthetic and systemic complications, including the risk to life.

In order to prevent SEG, we recommend the use of small-caliber cannulas and serial liposuction instead of megaliposuction.

The use of high-dose corticosteroids is the current approach to preventing the development of EMS.(52,53)

Pre-operative and early post-operative ambulation is recommended to prevent DVT and PTE. The use of epidural anesthesia, reducing surgical time and anesthesia time can be advantageous.

For high-risk patients, pneumatic compression devices may have more benefits than a continuous pressure device. Low doses of subcutaneous heparin (2500 U every 12 hours, starting 2 hours after the operation) reduce the incidence of DVT, but can also increase the risk of bleeding, preferably using fractionated heparin.(Fig. 5,6,7,8)

Liposuction: Recommendations

- Assess your general state of health and any pre-existing health conditions or risk factors;

- Taking photos for medical records;

- Discuss your options and recommend a treatment;

- Discuss the likely results of the surgery and any potential risks or complications.

1. Team with the surgeon

2. Preoperative:

Assess the patient, emphasizing previous reactions to local anesthetics, the presence of tachycardia with infiltrations for other procedures and determining the patient's exact weight.

Take special care with the following patients:

Hypertensive patients, patients with cardiovascular disease, a history suggestive of pheochromocytoma, hyperthyroidism, carcinoid tumors, those taking pseudoephedrine, antigripal and nutritional supplements with a product similar to ephedrine; all of these because of their greater susceptibility to exogenous catecholamines.

Diabetics have a higher risk of infection and poor healing, especially when they are not well controlled, as well as less tolerance to fluid loads according to their commitment to the target organ. Epilepsy and other seizure syndromes are very important to take into account, as it would be very difficult to determine whether they are convulsing during the procedure due to their underlying disease or the neurotoxicity of lidocaine.

It is important to premeditate with clonidine 0.075 mg, half a tablet, in patients without a history of bradycardia or hypotension. Be aware of the surgery to be performed and the volume to be extracted. Write in the patient's medical history the permitted doses of lidocaine according to the patient's weight.

3. In the intraoperative period:

Avoid multiple surgeries

When the procedure to be performed requires general anesthesia, inhalation anesthesia using isoflurane or sevoflurane. Halides such as desflurane or halothane will not be used due to their interaction with catecholamines. Hypnotic agents such as propofol and sodium thiopental are suitable for induction. Propofol, due to its half-life and metabolism, can be used as an infusion as a hypnotic component of a balanced anesthetic.

Any of the new opioids can be used to induce anesthesia. Especially those with short half-lives, such as remifentanil and alfentanil. Remifentanil, due to its plasma metabolism and ultra-short half-life, is a good option for maintaining balanced anesthesia.

The use of benzodiazepines should be avoided as much as possible due to their sedative and hypnotic characteristics and their pharmacological interaction at the level of cytochrome P 450 with local anesthetics. If co-interaction is necessary, the alternative is midazolam.

In general terms, the use of muscle relaxants is not routinely necessary in this type of surgery. If necessary, those with a short and intermediate half-life will be chosen. These will be reinforced by high doses of local anesthetics.

Our recommendation is balanced anesthesia with Remifentanil and Isofluoran.

It is important to use the solutions:

1. Know this. Always use the same presentation of the local anesthetic to make the dilutions, lidocaine 1%.

2. Clearly label the concentrations of the solutions to be used in milligrams per liter.

3. Prepare the dilutions the same day, before the procedure.

4. Use normal saline solution (0.9%) as a solvent.

5. Preparation of solutions by certified personnel

6. Standardization of the infiltration technique

During the postoperative period, careful monitoring of the patient should be taken in terms of state of consciousness, hemodynamic stability, pain management. Do not use sedatives during the first 24 hours of postoperative barbiturates, benzodiazepines, opioids and anti-histamines. When using general anesthesia, don't put Lidocaine in tumescent solutions.(54).

Conclusion:

Liposuction is a highly effective procedure. However, there are risks inherent in the surgical procedure that increasingly need to be studied and better understood. This survey of the MEDLINE/PubMed database selected 54 articles of interest dealing with complications of liposuction for aesthetic purposes only.

Among the complications reported in the articles, a noteworthy one is fat embolism, which has also been demonstrated in experimental studies and should therefore be increasingly suspected, as there is a relatively high incidence after liposuction, whether or not associated with lipografting. The literature reviewed warns of this potential risk; in addition, there are several other case reports of patients who developed respiratory discomfort as a result of pulmonary fat embolism.

The incidence of complications resulting from fat embolism in humans is still low, probably due to a lack of studies or even the difficulty in diagnosing it, especially in cases with little obvious clinical repercussions. Greater attention is needed in the post-operative period of liposuction surgeries in humans, with greater commitment from the doctors who carry out this procedure. Furthermore, when diagnosed, these cases should be published in the relevant medical literature, because only then will it be possible to establish the real incidence and complications of fat mobilization, which has been very evident in several experimental studies (10,14,18,21). Further studies with an emphasis on clinical importance are needed, as well as experimental research and clinical studies on this controversial subject, which is of great interest to society and especially to surgeons working in this area.

As the population is young and, in most cases, healthy, little morbidity and even less mortality is expected during and after any type of surgical procedure, such as liposuction.

Table 1

PROFOUND VENOUS THROMBOSIS	RISK FACTORS	RECOMMENDATIONS
BAJO RISK	- _ [40 years - I don't use oral contraceptives or hormone therapy. - Not chronic illness, malignancy or infection. - No family history - There is no history, no insufficiency venous.	-Comfortable position on the operating table -Knee flexion -Walking at the start of compression -Medium post-graduation.
MODERATE RISK	-] 40 years old - Use of oral contraceptives or hormone therapy Chronic, malignant or infectious disease - Family history - Short procedure Compulsive abdominal gynecological surgery	- Same as low-risk intermittent pneumatic compression . --Table position exchange or-Heparin 5000uc / 12h -HBPM 20mg / day 24h post-op . - As well as low risk - hematology
HIGH RISK	- Any age with prolonged procedure. -History of hormone use -History of chronic malignant or infectious disease -Background family	pre-surgical intra-histography with ant. previous - Consider pre-surgical use heparin 500u / 8h or BPM 40MG C / 12H - intermittent pneumatic compression and frequent change the intra-operative position

Table 2

Volume ratio of infiltrated liquids versus blood loss

	INFILTRATION	**BLOOD LOSS**
Dry technique	No.	20-25% (45,46)
Wet technique	200-300cc / area	4-30% (40,45)
Super-wet technique	1 cc infiltrated: 1 cc aspirated 3cc	1% (44)
Tumescent technique	infiltrated: 1 cc aspirated	1% (41,47,48)

Fig. 1 A. Abdominal liposuction procedure.

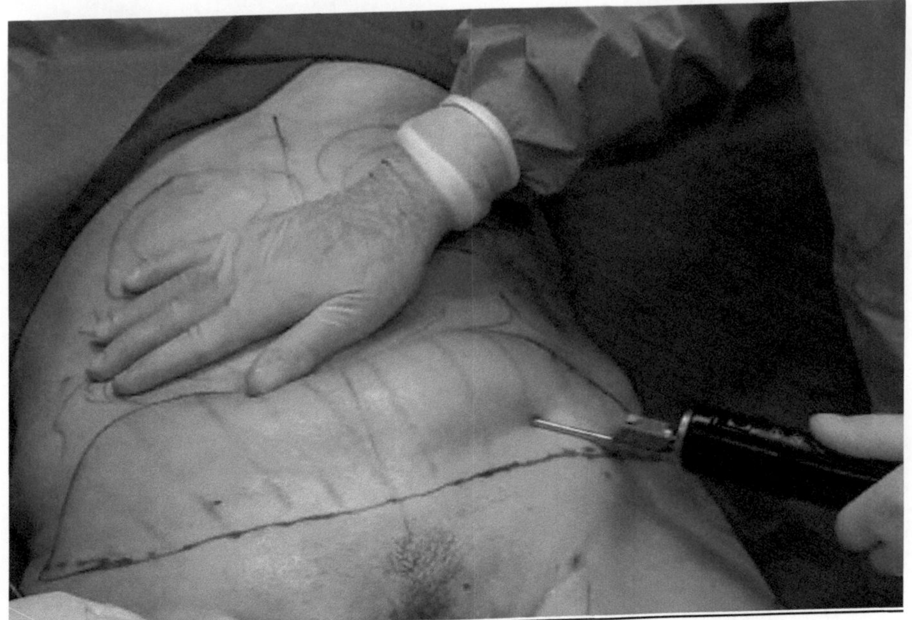

Fig. 1 B. Abdominal liposuction procedure.

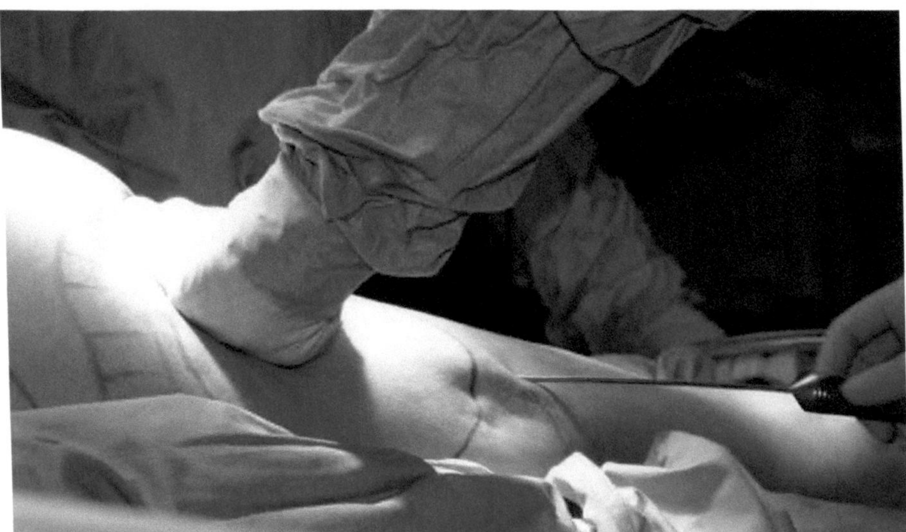

<u>Fig. 2.</u> Thigh liposuction procedure

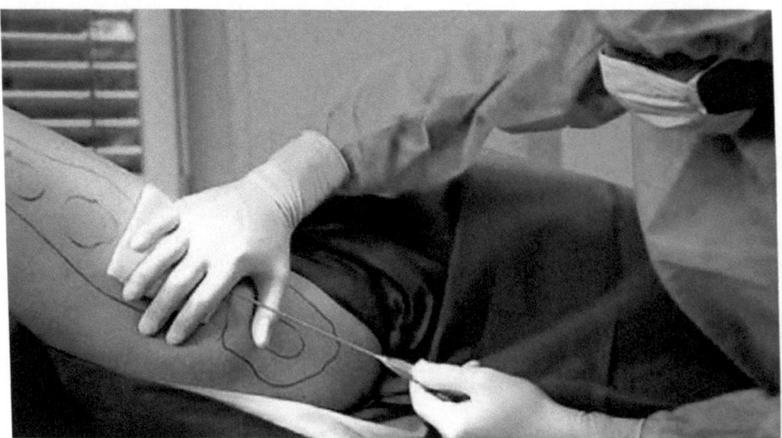

 Marking regions for liposuction procedures.

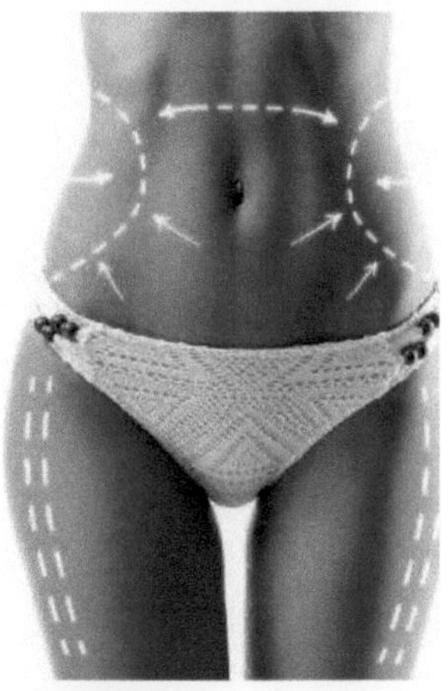

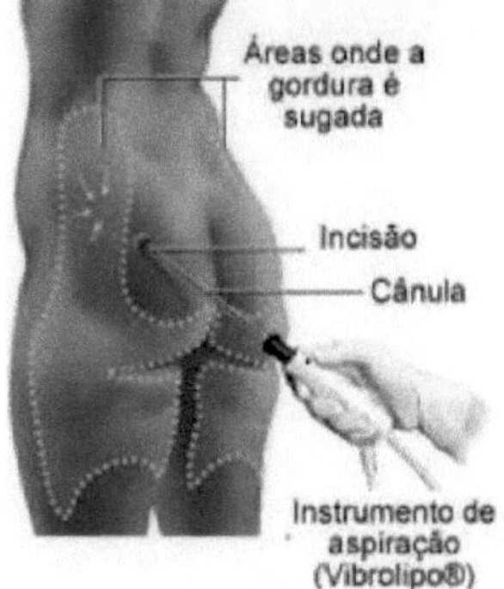

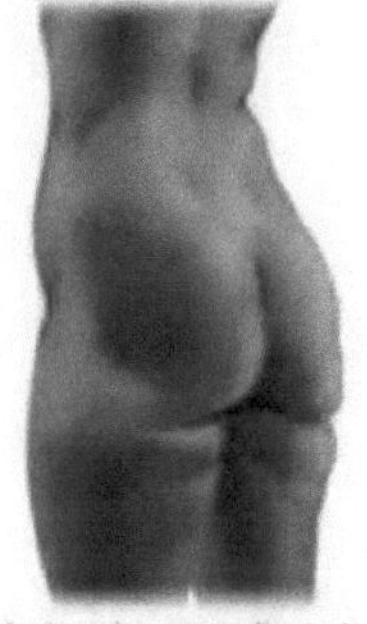
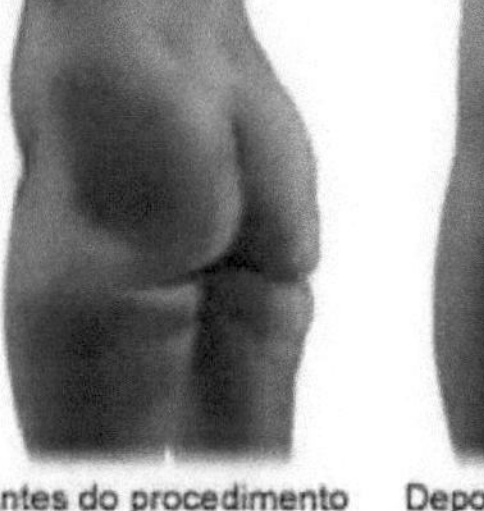

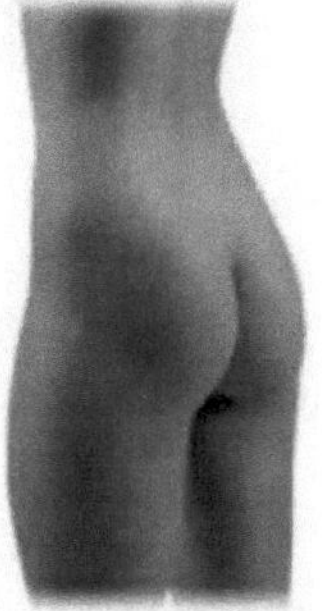

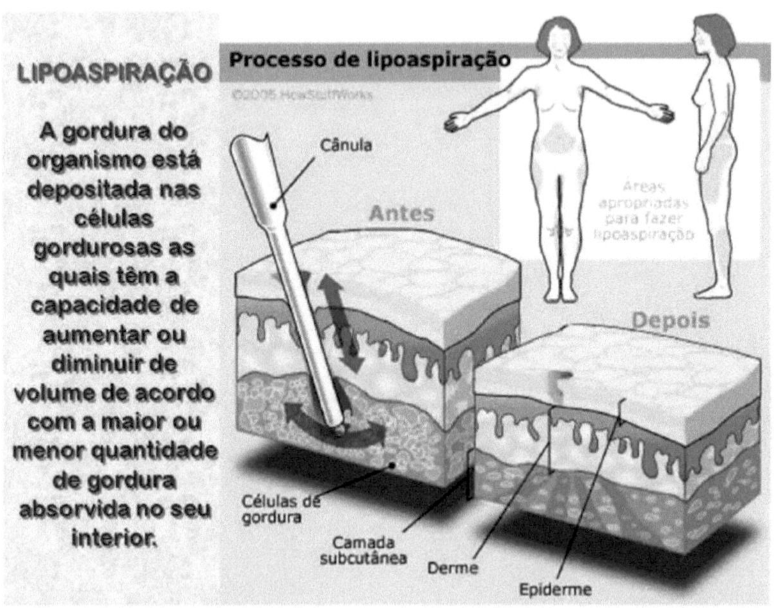

Fig. 4 B. Liposuction process.

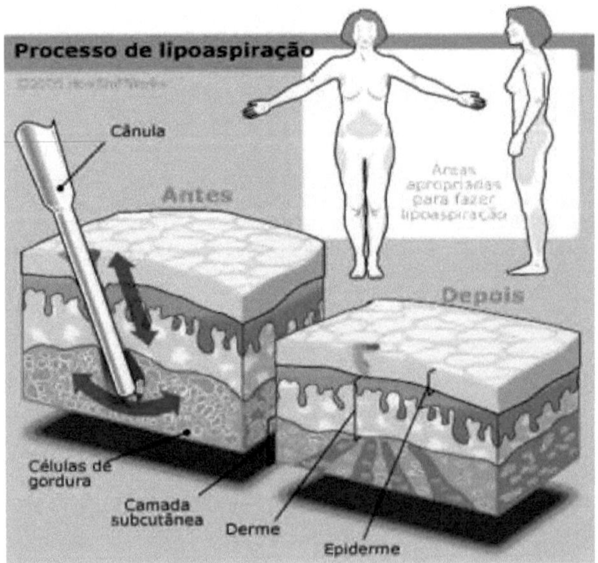

Fig. 5 Safety in the liposuction procedure

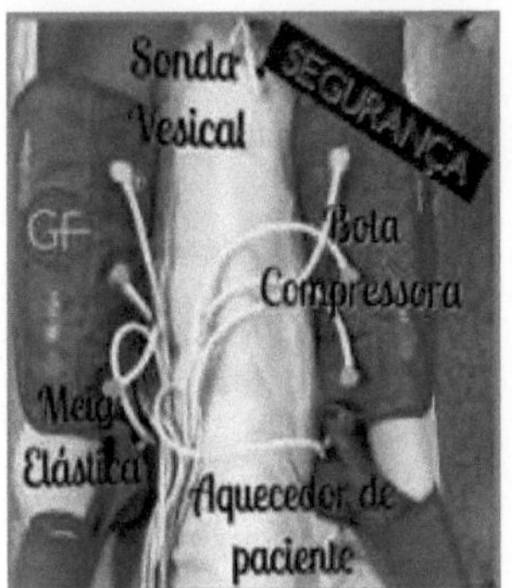

Fig. 6 - Standing flexion during surgery to activate calf muscles in cases where intermittent compression devices cannot be used.

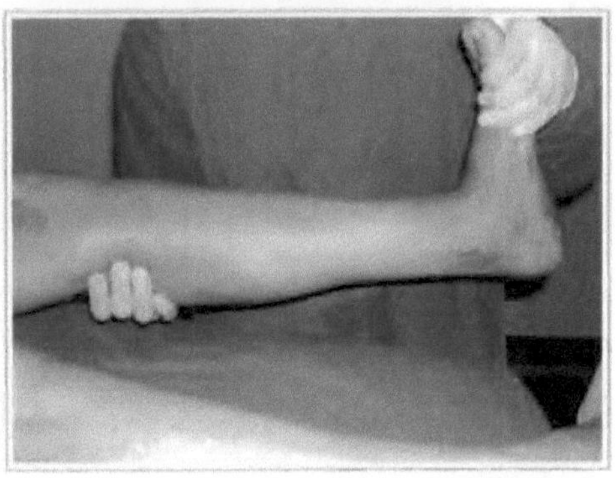

Fig. 7 - Use of a pneumatic compression device on the lower limbs.

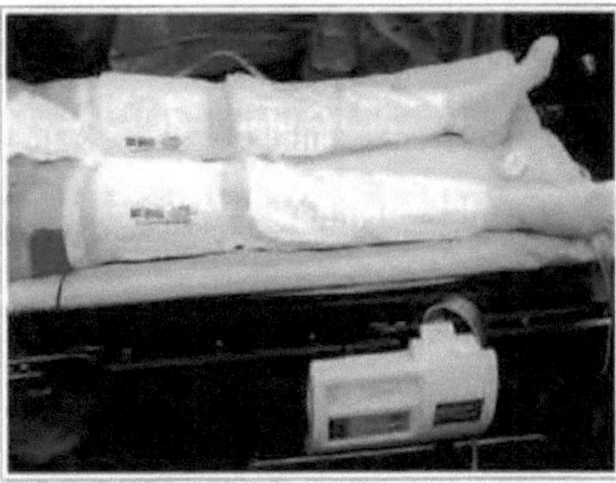

Fig. 8 - Elastic stocking with pressure graduation

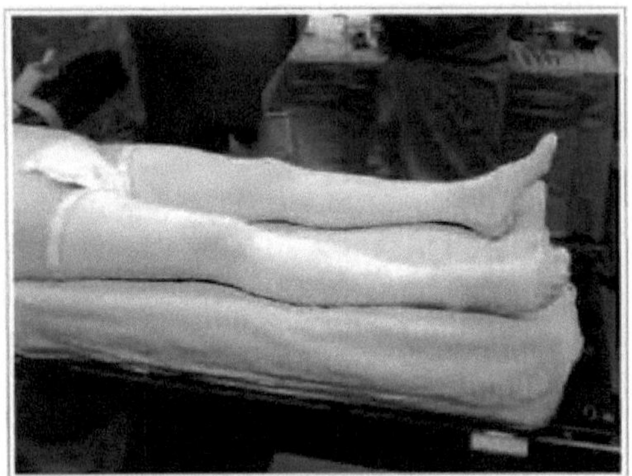

Bibliographical references:

1. Coleman, WP. The history of Liposuction and fat transplantation in America. Dermatol Clin 17: 723 - 730, 1999

2. Illouz. Y.G.: History and current concepts in lipoplasty. Clinics in plastic surgery. 25; 4: 721- 730, 1999

3. Gingrass, M.: Lipoplasty complications and their prevention. Clinics in plastic surgery 26; 3: 341 -354, 1999

4. Hanke, W. : Morbidity and mortality related to liposuction. Questions and answers. Dermatol Clin 17: 4 Oct 1999

5. Teimourian, B. : Complications associated with suction lipectomy. Clinics in plastic surgery. 16: 385, 1989

6. Basic Histology I L.C. Junqueira and José Carneiro. - 12 . ed]. - Rio de Janeiro: Guanabara Koogan, 2013.

7. Abraham L. Kierszenbaum. Histology and Cell Biology, An Introduction to Pathology. 3ª edition. Elsevier, 2012

8. Hernadez F Carvalho, Carla Beatriz Collares Buzato. Cells: A multidisciplinary approach. Manole Publishing House, 2005

9. Ovrebo, K.K., Grong, K. : Small intestinal perforation and peritonitis after abdominal suction lipoplasty. Ann. Plast. Surg, 38: 642 - 644, 1997.

10. Teimourian B, Rogers, W.B.: A national survey of complications associated with suction lipectomy: A comparative study. Plast. Reconstr. Surg. 84: 628 - 631, 1989.

11. Fredricks S. Analysis and introduction of a technology: Ultrasound assisted lipoplasty Task Force. Clin. Plast. Surg. 1999; 26 (2).

12. Hull RD, Pineo. Medical Clinics of North America. 1998; 82 (3).

13. Bick RL, Haas S. Medical Clinics of North America. 1998; 82 (3).

14. Schnur PL. Deep Vein Thrombosis Prophylaxis. Plast. Reconst. Surg. 1999; 6: 1923-28.

15. Claget GP, Anderson FA. Prevention of Venous Thromboembolism. Chest 1998; 114: 531S-560S.

16. Courtiss, E et al.: Large volume suction lipectomy: An analysis of 108 patients. Plastic

and reconstructive surgery. June 1992

17. Evaldo A. D'Assumpçâo, Luiz Pimentel, Rolf Gemperli, Ricardo Baroudi. Debate - Year 2005 - Volume 20 - Number 2.

18. Ross RM, Johnson GW. Fat embolism and the fat embolism syndrome. A double-blind therapeutic study. J. Bone Joint Surg. 1987; 69:128-131.

19. Kessler C. Low molecular weight heparins: Practical considerations. Seminars in hematology. 1997; 34 (4): 35-42

20. Kakkar V. Low molecular weight heparins: Prophylaxis of Venous Thromboembolism in Surgical Patients. Seminars in hematology. 1997; 34 (4): 9-19.

21. Schonfeld SA, Ploysongsang Y. Fat embolism prophylaxis with corticosteroids. Aprospective study in high-risk patients. Ann. Intern. Med. 1983; 99:438-443.

22. Fodor P. Wetting Solutions in Ultrasound Assisted Lipoplasty. Clin Plast Surg. Vol 26 N 2. 1999

23. Butterwick K, Goldman MP: Lidocaine Levels During the First Two Hours of Infiltration of Dilute Anesthetic Solution for Tumescent Liposuction: Rapid versus Slow Delivery. Dermatol Surg 25: 681-685. 1999.

24. Burk RE, Guzman-Stein G, Vasconez LO: Lidocain and Epinephrine levels in Tumescent Technique Liposuction. Plast Reconstr Surg 97:1379-1384. 1996.

25. Manson JE, Faich GA: Pharmacotherapy for Obesity -Do the Benefits outweigh the Risks? N Engl J Med 335:659-660.

26. Perry AW, Petti C, Rankin M: Lidocaine is not Necessary in Lipoplasty. Plast Reconstr Surg 104:1900-1906,1999

27. Klein JA: Anesthetic Formulation of Tumescent Solutions. Dermatol Clin 17:751-759. 1999

28. Klein JA, Kassarjdian N: Lidocaine Toxicity with Tumescent Liposuction. Dermatol Surg 23: 1169-1174. 1997.

29. Forman HP, Levin S, Stewart B: Cerebral Vasculitis and Hemorrhage in an Adolescent Taking Diet Pills Containing Phenylpropanolamine. Pediatrics 83:737-741,1989.

30. H Wen PY, Feske S, Theoh S: Cerebral Hemorrhage in a Patient Taking Fenfluramine and Phentermine for Obesity. Neurology 49:632-633. 199726.

31. Rohrich RJ, Beran SJ: Is Liposuction Safe? Plast Reconstr Surg 104:819822,1999.

32. Hetter G. Closed Suction Lipoplasty on 1078 patients: Illouz told the truth. Aesth. Plast. Surg. 1.988. 12: 183-187

33. Grazer F. Suction assisted lipectomy, suction lipectomy, lipolysis and lipexeresis. Plast. Reconstr.Surg. 1.983. 72: 620-624.

34. Courtiss E. Suction lipectomy: A retrospective analysis of 100 patients. 1.984. 73: 780-785.

35. Pitman G, Holzer J. Safe suction: fluid replacement and blood loss parameters. Perspect. Plast. Surg. 1.991. 5(1):81-89.

36. Latrenta, GS. Suction-Assisted Lipectomy. En: Rees TD, Latrenta GS. Aesthetic Plastic Surgery. 2ª . Edición. Philadelphia, PA. 1179-1241.

37. Latrenta, GS. Suction-Assisted Lipectomy. En: Rees TD, Latrenta GS. Aesthetic Plastic Surgery. 2nd Edition. Philadelphia, PA. 1179-1241.

38. Goodpasture J, Bunkis, J. Quantitative Analysis of Blood and Fat in Suction Lipectomy Aspirates. Plastic and Reconstructive Surgery. 1.986. 765-772.

39. SamdaL, F. Blood Loss During Liposuction Using the Tumescent Technique. Aesth. Plast. Surg. 1.994. 18: 157-160.8.

40. Pitman, G. Et al. Tumescent Liposuction. A Surgeon's perspective. Clin.Plast. Surg. April 1.996

41. Hetter, G. Blood and Fluid Replacement for Lipoplasty Procedures. Clin. Plast. Surg.1.989. 16(2). 245-247.

42. Rohrich RJ, Beran SJ, Bela Fodor P. The role of Subcutaneous Infiltration in Suction-Assisted Lipoplasty: A review. Plast. Reconstr. Surg. 1.997. 99(2). 526.

43. Clayton DN, Clayton JN, Lindley TS, ClaytoN JL. Large Volume Lipoplasty. Clin. Plast. Surg. 1.989. 16(2). 305-312.

44. Courtiss EH, Choucair RJ, Donelan MB. Large-Volume Suction Lipectomy: An Analysis of 108 patients. Plast. Reconstr. Surg. 1.992. 89(6) 1068-1079.

45. Klein JA. The tumescent technique. Dermatol. Clin. 1.990.8(3). 425-434.

46. Klein ja. Tumescent Technique for local anesthesia improves safety in large volume liposuction. Plast. Reconstr. Surg. 1.993. 92(6). 1085-1098.

47. Klein JA: Tumescent Technique for Local Anaesthesia Improves Safety in Large Volume Liposuction. Plast Reconstr Surg 92:1085-1098. 1993

48. Gingrass MK. Lipoplasty Complications and Their Prevention. Clin. Plast. Surg. 26(3). 341-354.

49. Gilliland MD, Coates N. Tumescent Liposuction complicated by Pulmonary Edema. Plast. Reconst. Surg. 1.997. 99(1). 215-219.

50. Hiyama DT, Zinner MJ. Surgical Complications. En: Schwartz SI et al. Principles of Surgery. 6ª . Edición. USA. 464-466.

51. Fein, A. Et al. Pulmonary edema fluid Studies. Critical Care Clinics. July, 1986. 446-447.

52. Kirby R. Perioperative Fluid Therapy and Postoperative Pulmonary Edema. Cause-Effect Relationship? CHEST. 1.999. 115(5) May.1224-1226.

53. Trott SA, Beran SJ, Rohrich RJ. Et al. Safety Considerations and Fluid Resuscitation in Liposuction: An Analysis of 53 Consecutive Patients. Plast Reconst. Surg. 1.998. 102(6). 2220-2229.

54. Tsay RY, Lai CH, Chan HL. Evaluation of blood loss during tumescent liposuction in Orientals, Dermatologic Surgery - 1998 Dec; 24 (12): 1326-9

55. Klein J. Anesthetic formulation of tumescent solutions, Clinicas Dermatológicas, vol.17, No4, 1999, pg 751.

56. Hanke W., Coleman W. Morbidity and Mortality Related to Liposuction, Clinicas Dematológicas, vol. 17, No4, 1999, pg 899.

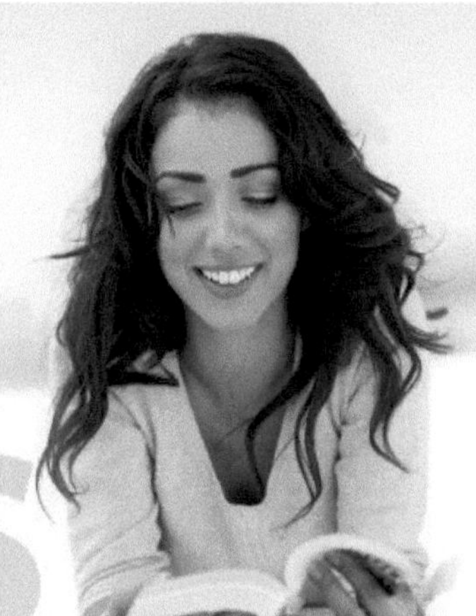

I want morebooks!

Buy your books fast and straightforward online - at one of world's fastest growing online book stores! Environmentally sound due to Print-on-Demand technologies.

Buy your books online at
www.morebooks.shop

Kaufen Sie Ihre Bücher schnell und unkompliziert online – auf einer der am schnellsten wachsenden Buchhandelsplattformen weltweit! Dank Print-On-Demand umwelt- und ressourcenschonend produziert.

Bücher schneller online kaufen
www.morebooks.shop

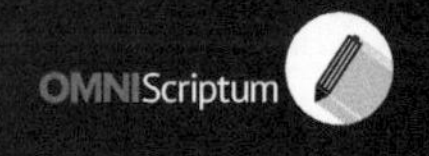

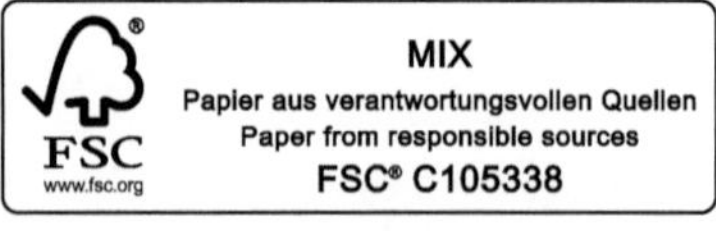

Printed by Books on Demand GmbH, Norderstedt / Germany